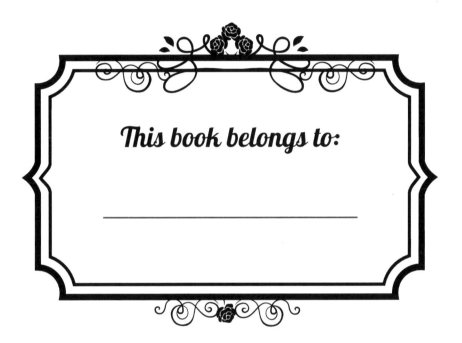

This book belongs to:

_____

DATE	# WEEK

NAME	🌱 DOSAGE	💊 TIME
		: ⠀⠀⠀⠀ AM / PM
		: ⠀⠀⠀⠀ AM / PM
		: ⠀⠀⠀⠀ AM / PM
		: ⠀⠀⠀⠀ AM / PM
		: ⠀⠀⠀⠀ AM / PM
		: ⠀⠀⠀⠀ AM / PM
		: ⠀⠀⠀⠀ AM / PM
		: ⠀⠀⠀⠀ AM / PM
		: ⠀⠀⠀⠀ AM / PM
		: ⠀⠀⠀⠀ AM / PM
		: ⠀⠀⠀⠀ AM / PM
		: ⠀⠀⠀⠀ AM / PM
		: ⠀⠀⠀⠀ AM / PM
		: ⠀⠀⠀⠀ AM / PM
		: ⠀⠀⠀⠀ AM / PM

SIDE EFFECTS	📝 ADDITIONAL NOTES

PHYSICAL CONDITION

SLEEP		🥛 WATER	
ENERGY		🏃 ACTIVITY	

📅 DATE		# WEEK

💊 NAME	🌱 DOSAGE	🕐 TIME
		: AM
		: AM
		: AM
		: AM
		: AM
		: AM
		: AM
		: AM
		: AM
		: AM
		: AM
		: AM
		: AM
		: AM
		: AM

🧠 SIDE EFFECTS	📝 ADDITIONAL NOTES
•	
•	
•	
•	
•	

PHYSICAL CONDITION	
🌙 SLEEP	💧 WATER
⚡ ENERGY	🏃 ACTIVITY

DATE	# WEEK	

NAME	🌱 DOSAGE	⏰ TIME
		: AM / PM
		: AM / PM
		: AM / PM
		: AM / PM
		: AM / PM
		: AM / PM
		: AM / PM
		: AM / PM
		: AM / PM
		: AM / PM
		: AM / PM
		: AM / PM
		: AM / PM
		: AM / PM
		: AM / PM

SIDE EFFECTS

📝 **ADDITIONAL NOTES**

PHYSICAL CONDITION

SLEEP		🥛 WATER	
ENERGY		🏃 ACTIVITY	

📅 DATE		#️⃣ WEEK	

💊 NAME	🌱 DOSAGE	⏰ TIME	
		:	AM
		:	AM
		:	AM
		:	AM
		:	AM
		:	AM
		:	AM
		:	AM
		:	AM
		:	AM
		:	AM
		:	AM
		:	AM
		:	AM
		:	AM

🧠 SIDE EFFECTS

-
-
-
-
-

📝 ADDITIONAL NOTES

PHYSICAL CONDITION

🌙 SLEEP		💧 WATER	
⚡ ENERGY		🏃 ACTIVITY	

DATE	# WEEK

NAME	DOSAGE	TIME
		: AM / PM
		: AM / PM
		: AM / PM
		: AM / PM
		: AM / PM
		: AM / PM
		: AM / PM
		: AM / PM
		: AM / PM
		: AM / PM
		: AM / PM
		: AM / PM
		: AM / PM
		: AM / PM
		: AM / PM

SIDE EFFECTS

ADDITIONAL NOTES

PHYSICAL CONDITION	
SLEEP	WATER
ENERGY	ACTIVITY

🗓 DATE		# WEEK

💊 NAME	🌱 DOSAGE	💊 TIME
		: AM
		: AM
		: AM
		: AM
		: AM
		: AM
		: AM
		: AM
		: AM
		: AM
		: AM
		: AM
		: AM
		: AM
		: AM

🧠 SIDE EFFECTS	📝 ADDITIONAL NOTES
•	
•	
•	
•	
•	

PHYSICAL CONDITION			
🌙 SLEEP		🥛 WATER	
⚡ ENERGY		🏃 ACTIVITY	

DATE	# WEEK	

NAME	🌱 DOSAGE	⏰ TIME
		: AM / PM
		: AM / PM
		: AM / PM
		: AM / PM
		: AM / PM
		: AM / PM
		: AM / PM
		: AM / PM
		: AM / PM
		: AM / PM
		: AM / PM
		: AM / PM
		: AM / PM
		: AM / PM
		: AM / PM

SIDE EFFECTS

📝 ADDITIONAL NOTES

PHYSICAL CONDITION

SLEEP	🔲🔲🔲🔲	💧 WATER	🔲🔲🔲🔲
ENERGY	🔲🔲🔲🔲	🏃 ACTIVITY	🔲🔲🔲🔲

📅 DATE			#️⃣ WEEK	

💊 NAME	🌱 DOSAGE	⏰ TIME
		: AM
		: AM
		: AM
		: AM
		: AM
		: AM
		: AM
		: AM
		: AM
		: AM
		: AM
		: AM
		: AM
		: AM
		: AM

🧠 SIDE EFFECTS	📝 ADDITIONAL NOTES
•	
•	
•	
•	
•	

PHYSICAL CONDITION	
🌙 SLEEP	💧 WATER
⚡ ENERGY	🏃 ACTIVITY

DATE	# WEEK

NAME	🪴 DOSAGE	🍥 TIME
		: AM / PM
		: AM / PM
		: AM / PM
		: AM / PM
		: AM / PM
		: AM / PM
		: AM / PM
		: AM / PM
		: AM / PM
		: AM / PM
		: AM / PM
		: AM / PM
		: AM / PM
		: AM / PM
		: AM / PM

SIDE EFFECTS	📝 ADDITIONAL NOTES

PHYSICAL CONDITION

SLEEP		WATER	
ENERGY		🏃 ACTIVITY	

📅 DATE		#️⃣ WEEK

💊 NAME	🌱 DOSAGE	🕐 TIME
		: AM
		: AM
		: AM
		: AM
		: AM
		: AM
		: AM
		: AM
		: AM
		: AM
		: AM
		: AM
		: AM
		: AM
		: AM

🧠 SIDE EFFECTS

-
-
-
-
-

📝 ADDITIONAL NOTES

PHYSICAL CONDITION

🌙 SLEEP		🥤 WATER	
🔆 ENERGY		🏃 ACTIVITY	

DATE	#️ WEEK	

NAME	🌱 DOSAGE	🕐 TIME
		: AM / PM
		: AM / PM
		: AM / PM
		: AM / PM
		: AM / PM
		: AM / PM
		: AM / PM
		: AM / PM
		: AM / PM
		: AM / PM
		: AM / PM
		: AM / PM
		: AM / PM
		: AM / PM
		: AM / PM

SIDE EFFECTS	📝 ADDITIONAL NOTES

PHYSICAL CONDITION

SLEEP		🥛 WATER	
ENERGY		🏃 ACTIVITY	

▦ DATE		# WEEK

℞ NAME	✿ DOSAGE	⏱ TIME
		: AM
		: AM
		: AM
		: AM
		: AM
		: AM
		: AM
		: AM
		: AM
		: AM
		: AM
		: AM
		: AM
		: AM
		: AM

🗠 SIDE EFFECTS

-
-
-
-
-

🗒 ADDITIONAL NOTES

PHYSICAL CONDITION

🌙 SLEEP		🥛 WATER	
⚡ ENERGY		🏃 ACTIVITY	

DATE		# WEEK	

NAME	DOSAGE	TIME	
		:	AM / PM
		:	AM / PM
		:	AM / PM
		:	AM / PM
		:	AM / PM
		:	AM / PM
		:	AM / PM
		:	AM / PM
		:	AM / PM
		:	AM / PM
		:	AM / PM
		:	AM / PM
		:	AM / PM
		:	AM / PM
		:	AM / PM

SIDE EFFECTS	ADDITIONAL NOTES

PHYSICAL CONDITION

SLEEP		WATER	
ENERGY		ACTIVITY	

📅 DATE		#️⃣ WEEK

💊 NAME	🌿 DOSAGE	⏱️ TIME
		: AM
		: AM
		: AM
		: AM
		: AM
		: AM
		: AM
		: AM
		: AM
		: AM
		: AM
		: AM
		: AM
		: AM
		: AM

🧠 SIDE EFFECTS

-
-
-
-
-

📝 ADDITIONAL NOTES

PHYSICAL CONDITION

🌙 SLEEP		💧 WATER	
⚡ ENERGY		🏃 ACTIVITY	

DATE	# WEEK

NAME	🌱 DOSAGE	💊 TIME	
		:	AM / PM
		:	AM / PM
		:	AM / PM
		:	AM / PM
		:	AM / PM
		:	AM / PM
		:	AM / PM
		:	AM / PM
		:	AM / PM
		:	AM / PM
		:	AM / PM
		:	AM / PM
		:	AM / PM
		:	AM / PM
		:	AM / PM

SIDE EFFECTS	📝 ADDITIONAL NOTES

PHYSICAL CONDITION

SLEEP		💧 WATER	
ENERGY		🏃 ACTIVITY	

📅 DATE		#️⃣ WEEK	

💊 NAME	💊 DOSAGE	🕐 TIME	
		:	AM
		:	AM
		:	AM
		:	AM
		:	AM
		:	AM
		:	AM
		:	AM
		:	AM
		:	AM
		:	AM
		:	AM
		:	AM
		:	AM
		:	AM

🗣 SIDE EFFECTS	📝 ADDITIONAL NOTES
•	
•	
•	
•	
•	

PHYSICAL CONDITION			
🌙 SLEEP	▭▭▭▭▭	🥛 WATER	▭▭▭▭▭
⚡ ENERGY	▭▭▭▭▭	🏃 ACTIVITY	▭▭▭▭▭

DATE		# WEEK	

NAME	DOSAGE	TIME	
		:	AM / PM
		:	AM / PM
		:	AM / PM
		:	AM / PM
		:	AM / PM
		:	AM / PM
		:	AM / PM
		:	AM / PM
		:	AM / PM
		:	AM / PM
		:	AM / PM
		:	AM / PM
		:	AM / PM
		:	AM / PM
		:	AM / PM

SIDE EFFECTS

ADDITIONAL NOTES

PHYSICAL CONDITION

SLEEP		WATER	
ENERGY		ACTIVITY	

📅 DATE		#️⃣ WEEK	

💊 NAME	🌱 DOSAGE	⏰ TIME	
		:	AM
		:	AM
		:	AM
		:	AM
		:	AM
		:	AM
		:	AM
		:	AM
		:	AM
		:	AM
		:	AM
		:	AM
		:	AM
		:	AM
		:	AM

🧠 SIDE EFFECTS
-
-
-
-
-

📝 ADDITIONAL NOTES

PHYSICAL CONDITION

🌙 SLEEP		💧 WATER	
⚡ ENERGY		🏃 ACTIVITY	

DATE	# WEEK

NAME	🪴 DOSAGE	🕐 TIME	
		:	AM / PM
		:	AM / PM
		:	AM / PM
		:	AM / PM
		:	AM / PM
		:	AM / PM
		:	AM / PM
		:	AM / PM
		:	AM / PM
		:	AM / PM
		:	AM / PM
		:	AM / PM
		:	AM / PM
		:	AM / PM
		:	AM / PM

SIDE EFFECTS	📝 ADDITIONAL NOTES

PHYSICAL CONDITION

SLEEP		WATER	
ENERGY		ACTIVITY	

📅 DATE		#️⃣ WEEK

💊 NAME	🪴 DOSAGE	⏰ TIME
		: AM
		: AM
		: AM
		: AM
		: AM
		: AM
		: AM
		: AM
		: AM
		: AM
		: AM
		: AM
		: AM
		: AM
		: AM

🧠 SIDE EFFECTS

-
-
-
-
-

📝 ADDITIONAL NOTES

PHYSICAL CONDITION

🌙 SLEEP		💧 WATER	
⚡ ENERGY		🏃 ACTIVITY	

DATE		# WEEK	

NAME	🌱 DOSAGE	⏰ TIME	
		:	AM / PM
		:	AM / PM
		:	AM / PM
		:	AM / PM
		:	AM / PM
		:	AM / PM
		:	AM / PM
		:	AM / PM
		:	AM / PM
		:	AM / PM
		:	AM / PM
		:	AM / PM
		:	AM / PM
		:	AM / PM
		:	AM / PM

SIDE EFFECTS

📝 ADDITIONAL NOTES

PHYSICAL CONDITION

SLEEP		🥛 WATER	
ENERGY		🏃 ACTIVITY	

📅 DATE		# WEEK

💊 NAME	🌱 DOSAGE	⏰ TIME
		: AM
		: AM
		: AM
		: AM
		: AM
		: AM
		: AM
		: AM
		: AM
		: AM
		: AM
		: AM
		: AM
		: AM

🧠 SIDE EFFECTS

-
-
-
-
-

📝 ADDITIONAL NOTES

PHYSICAL CONDITION

🌙 SLEEP		💧 WATER	
⚡ ENERGY		🏃 ACTIVITY	

DATE	#️ WEEK

NAME	🌱 DOSAGE	⏰ TIME	
		:	AM / PM
		:	AM / PM
		:	AM / PM
		:	AM / PM
		:	AM / PM
		:	AM / PM
		:	AM / PM
		:	AM / PM
		:	AM / PM
		:	AM / PM
		:	AM / PM
		:	AM / PM
		:	AM / PM
		:	AM / PM
		:	AM / PM

SIDE EFFECTS	📝 ADDITIONAL NOTES

PHYSICAL CONDITION

SLEEP	WATER
ENERGY	🏃 ACTIVITY

📅 DATE		#️⃣ WEEK

💊 NAME	🌱 DOSAGE	⏰ TIME
		: AM
		: AM
		: AM
		: AM
		: AM
		: AM
		: AM
		: AM
		: AM
		: AM
		: AM
		: AM
		: AM
		: AM
		: AM

🧠 SIDE EFFECTS

-
-
-
-
-

📝 ADDITIONAL NOTES

PHYSICAL CONDITION

🌙 SLEEP		🥤 WATER	
⚡ ENERGY		🏃 ACTIVITY	

DATE	🗓 WEEK

NAME	🪴 DOSAGE	🕐 TIME
		: AM / PM
		: AM / PM
		: AM / PM
		: AM / PM
		: AM / PM
		: AM / PM
		: AM / PM
		: AM / PM
		: AM / PM
		: AM / PM
		: AM / PM
		: AM / PM
		: AM / PM
		: AM / PM

SIDE EFFECTS

📝 ADDITIONAL NOTES

PHYSICAL CONDITION

SLEEP		🥛 WATER	
ENERGY		🏃 ACTIVITY	

📅 DATE		# WEEK

💊 NAME	🌱 DOSAGE	💊 TIME
		: AM
		: AM
		: AM
		: AM
		: AM
		: AM
		: AM
		: AM
		: AM
		: AM
		: AM
		: AM
		: AM
		: AM
		: AM

🧠 SIDE EFFECTS

-
-
-
-
-

📝 ADDITIONAL NOTES

PHYSICAL CONDITION

🌙 SLEEP		🥛 WATER	
⚡ ENERGY		🏃 ACTIVITY	

DATE	# WEEK	

NAME	🪴 DOSAGE	🕐 TIME
		: AM / PM
		: AM / PM
		: AM / PM
		: AM / PM
		: AM / PM
		: AM / PM
		: AM / PM
		: AM / PM
		: AM / PM
		: AM / PM
		: AM / PM
		: AM / PM
		: AM / PM
		: AM / PM
		: AM / PM

SIDE EFFECTS

📝 ADDITIONAL NOTES

PHYSICAL CONDITION

SLEEP	[			]	🥛 WATER	[			]
ENERGY	[			]	🏃 ACTIVITY	[			]

📅 DATE		#️⃣ WEEK

💊 NAME	🌱 DOSAGE	⏰ TIME
		: AM
		: AM
		: AM
		: AM
		: AM
		: AM
		: AM
		: AM
		: AM
		: AM
		: AM
		: AM
		: AM
		: AM
		: AM

🧠 SIDE EFFECTS	📝 ADDITIONAL NOTES
•	
•	
•	
•	
•	

PHYSICAL CONDITION	
🌙 SLEEP	💧 WATER
⚡ ENERGY	🏃 ACTIVITY

DATE	# WEEK

NAME	DOSAGE	TIME
		: AM / PM
		: AM / PM
		: AM / PM
		: AM / PM
		: AM / PM
		: AM / PM
		: AM / PM
		: AM / PM
		: AM / PM
		: AM / PM
		: AM / PM
		: AM / PM
		: AM / PM
		: AM / PM
		: AM / PM

SIDE EFFECTS	ADDITIONAL NOTES

PHYSICAL CONDITION

SLEEP		WATER	
ENERGY		ACTIVITY	

📅 DATE		#️⃣ WEEK

💊 NAME	🪴 DOSAGE	⏲️ TIME
		: AM
		: AM
		: AM
		: AM
		: AM
		: AM
		: AM
		: AM
		: AM
		: AM
		: AM
		: AM
		: AM
		: AM
		: AM

🧠 SIDE EFFECTS	📝 ADDITIONAL NOTES
•	
•	
•	
•	
•	

PHYSICAL CONDITION

🌙 SLEEP		🥛 WATER	
⚡ ENERGY		🏃 ACTIVITY	

DATE	# WEEK

NAME	🌱 DOSAGE	💊 TIME
		: AM / PM
		: AM / PM
		: AM / PM
		: AM / PM
		: AM / PM
		: AM / PM
		: AM / PM
		: AM / PM
		: AM / PM
		: AM / PM
		: AM / PM
		: AM / PM
		: AM / PM
		: AM / PM
		: AM / PM

SIDE EFFECTS

📝 ADDITIONAL NOTES

PHYSICAL CONDITION

SLEEP		🥛 WATER	
ENERGY		🏃 ACTIVITY	

📅 DATE		#️⃣ WEEK

💊 NAME	🪴 DOSAGE	⏰ TIME
		: AM
		: AM
		: AM
		: AM
		: AM
		: AM
		: AM
		: AM
		: AM
		: AM
		: AM
		: AM
		: AM
		: AM
		: AM

🧠 SIDE EFFECTS

-
-
-
-
-

📝 ADDITIONAL NOTES

PHYSICAL CONDITION

🌙 SLEEP		💧 WATER	
⚡ ENERGY		🏃 ACTIVITY	

DATE		▦ WEEK	

NAME	⚘ DOSAGE	⏱ TIME	
		:	AM / PM
		:	AM / PM
		:	AM / PM
		:	AM / PM
		:	AM / PM
		:	AM / PM
		:	AM / PM
		:	AM / PM
		:	AM / PM
		:	AM / PM
		:	AM / PM
		:	AM / PM
		:	AM / PM
		:	AM / PM
		:	AM / PM

SIDE EFFECTS	📝 ADDITIONAL NOTES

PHYSICAL CONDITION

SLEEP	⬭⬭⬭⬭⬭	🥛 WATER	⬭⬭⬭⬭⬭
ENERGY	⬭⬭⬭⬭⬭	🏃 ACTIVITY	⬭⬭⬭⬭⬭

📅 DATE		# WEEK

💊 NAME	🌱 DOSAGE	🕐 TIME
		: AM
		: AM
		: AM
		: AM
		: AM
		: AM
		: AM
		: AM
		: AM
		: AM
		: AM
		: AM
		: AM
		: AM
		: AM

🧠 SIDE EFFECTS	📝 ADDITIONAL NOTES
•	
•	
•	
•	
•	

PHYSICAL CONDITION	
🌙 SLEEP	🥤 WATER
⚡ ENERGY	🏃 ACTIVITY

DATE		# WEEK	

NAME	DOSAGE	TIME	
		:	AM / PM
		:	AM / PM
		:	AM / PM
		:	AM / PM
		:	AM / PM
		:	AM / PM
		:	AM / PM
		:	AM / PM
		:	AM / PM
		:	AM / PM
		:	AM / PM
		:	AM / PM
		:	AM / PM
		:	AM / PM
		:	AM / PM

SIDE EFFECTS

ADDITIONAL NOTES

PHYSICAL CONDITION

SLEEP		WATER	
ENERGY		ACTIVITY	

📅 DATE		#️⃣ WEEK	

💊 NAME	🌱 DOSAGE	🕐 TIME	
		:	AM
		:	AM
		:	AM
		:	AM
		:	AM
		:	AM
		:	AM
		:	AM
		:	AM
		:	AM
		:	AM
		:	AM
		:	AM
		:	AM
		:	AM

🧠 SIDE EFFECTS	📝 ADDITIONAL NOTES
•	
•	
•	
•	
•	

PHYSICAL CONDITION	
🌙 SLEEP	🥛 WATER
⚡ ENERGY	🏃 ACTIVITY

DATE			# WEEK		

NAME	DOSAGE	TIME	
		:	AM / PM
		:	AM / PM
		:	AM / PM
		:	AM / PM
		:	AM / PM
		:	AM / PM
		:	AM / PM
		:	AM / PM
		:	AM / PM
		:	AM / PM
		:	AM / PM
		:	AM / PM
		:	AM / PM
		:	AM / PM
		:	AM / PM

SIDE EFFECTS

ADDITIONAL NOTES

PHYSICAL CONDITION

SLEEP		WATER	
ENERGY		ACTIVITY	

🗓 DATE		#️ WEEK

💊 NAME	🌱 DOSAGE	🕐 TIME
		: AM
		: AM
		: AM
		: AM
		: AM
		: AM
		: AM
		: AM
		: AM
		: AM
		: AM
		: AM
		: AM
		: AM
		: AM

🗣 SIDE EFFECTS

-
-
-
-
-

📝 ADDITIONAL NOTES

PHYSICAL CONDITION

🌙 SLEEP		💧 WATER	
🔋 ENERGY		🏃 ACTIVITY	

DATE		# WEEK	

NAME	DOSAGE	TIME	
		:	AM / PM
		:	AM / PM
		:	AM / PM
		:	AM / PM
		:	AM / PM
		:	AM / PM
		:	AM / PM
		:	AM / PM
		:	AM / PM
		:	AM / PM
		:	AM / PM
		:	AM / PM
		:	AM / PM
		:	AM / PM
		:	AM / PM

SIDE EFFECTS

ADDITIONAL NOTES

PHYSICAL CONDITION	
SLEEP	WATER
ENERGY	ACTIVITY

⊞ DATE			# WEEK	

💊 NAME	🌱 DOSAGE	💊 TIME
		: AM
		: AM
		: AM
		: AM
		: AM
		: AM
		: AM
		: AM
		: AM
		: AM
		: AM
		: AM
		: AM
		: AM
		: AM

🧠 SIDE EFFECTS	📝 ADDITIONAL NOTES
•	
•	
•	
•	
•	

PHYSICAL CONDITION

🌙 SLEEP		💧 WATER	
⚡ ENERGY		🏃 ACTIVITY	

DATE		# WEEK	

NAME	🌱 DOSAGE	⏰ TIME	
		:	AM / PM
		:	AM / PM
		:	AM / PM
		:	AM / PM
		:	AM / PM
		:	AM / PM
		:	AM / PM
		:	AM / PM
		:	AM / PM
		:	AM / PM
		:	AM / PM
		:	AM / PM
		:	AM / PM
		:	AM / PM
		:	AM / PM

SIDE EFFECTS	📝 ADDITIONAL NOTES

PHYSICAL CONDITION

SLEEP	⬡⬡⬡⬡⬡	🥤 WATER	⬡⬡⬡⬡⬡
ENERGY	⬡⬡⬡⬡⬡	🏃 ACTIVITY	⬡⬡⬡⬡⬡

📅 DATE		# WEEK

💊 NAME	🌱 DOSAGE	⏰ TIME
		: AM
		: AM
		: AM
		: AM
		: AM
		: AM
		: AM
		: AM
		: AM
		: AM
		: AM
		: AM
		: AM
		: AM
		: AM

🧠 SIDE EFFECTS	📝 ADDITIONAL NOTES
•	
•	
•	
•	
•	

PHYSICAL CONDITION	
🌙 SLEEP	💧 WATER
⚡ ENERGY	🏃 ACTIVITY

DATE	# WEEK	

NAME	🪴 DOSAGE	⏱ TIME
		: AM / PM
		: AM / PM
		: AM / PM
		: AM / PM
		: AM / PM
		: AM / PM
		: AM / PM
		: AM / PM
		: AM / PM
		: AM / PM
		: AM / PM
		: AM / PM
		: AM / PM
		: AM / PM
		: AM / PM
		: AM / PM

SIDE EFFECTS	📝 ADDITIONAL NOTES

PHYSICAL CONDITION

SLEEP	[ ][ ][ ][ ]	🥛 WATER	[ ][ ][ ][ ]
ENERGY	[ ][ ][ ][ ]	🏃 ACTIVITY	[ ][ ][ ][ ]

📅 DATE		#️⃣ WEEK

💊 NAME	🌱 DOSAGE	⏰ TIME
		: AM
		: AM
		: AM
		: AM
		: AM
		: AM
		: AM
		: AM
		: AM
		: AM
		: AM
		: AM
		: AM
		: AM
		: AM

🧠 SIDE EFFECTS

-
-
-
-
-

📝 ADDITIONAL NOTES

PHYSICAL CONDITION

🌙 SLEEP		💧 WATER	
⚡ ENERGY		🏃 ACTIVITY	

DATE	# WEEK

NAME	🌱 DOSAGE	🕐 TIME
		: AM / PM
		: AM / PM
		: AM / PM
		: AM / PM
		: AM / PM
		: AM / PM
		: AM / PM
		: AM / PM
		: AM / PM
		: AM / PM
		: AM / PM
		: AM / PM
		: AM / PM
		: AM / PM

SIDE EFFECTS	📝 ADDITIONAL NOTES

PHYSICAL CONDITION

SLEEP		🥛 WATER	
ENERGY		🏃 ACTIVITY	

📅 DATE		# WEEK

💊 NAME	💊 DOSAGE	🕐 TIME
		: AM
		: AM
		: AM
		: AM
		: AM
		: AM
		: AM
		: AM
		: AM
		: AM
		: AM
		: AM
		: AM
		: AM
		: AM

🧠 SIDE EFFECTS	📝 ADDITIONAL NOTES
•	
•	
•	
•	
•	

PHYSICAL CONDITION	
🌙 SLEEP	🥛 WATER
⚡ ENERGY	🏃 ACTIVITY

DATE		# WEEK	

NAME	🧪 DOSAGE	🕐 TIME	
		:	AM / PM
		:	AM / PM
		:	AM / PM
		:	AM / PM
		:	AM / PM
		:	AM / PM
		:	AM / PM
		:	AM / PM
		:	AM / PM
		:	AM / PM
		:	AM / PM
		:	AM / PM
		:	AM / PM
		:	AM / PM
		:	AM / PM

SIDE EFFECTS	📝 ADDITIONAL NOTES

PHYSICAL CONDITION	
SLEEP	WATER
ENERGY	ACTIVITY

📅 DATE		#️⃣ WEEK

💊 NAME	🌱 DOSAGE	⏰ TIME
		: AM
		: AM
		: AM
		: AM
		: AM
		: AM
		: AM
		: AM
		: AM
		: AM
		: AM
		: AM
		: AM
		: AM
		: AM

🧠 SIDE EFFECTS	📝 ADDITIONAL NOTES
•	
•	
•	
•	
•	

PHYSICAL CONDITION

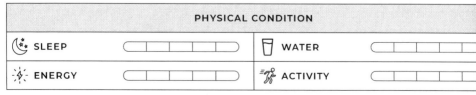

🌙 SLEEP   ▢▢▢▢▢   💧 WATER   ▢▢▢▢▢

⚡ ENERGY   ▢▢▢▢▢   🏃 ACTIVITY   ▢▢▢▢▢

DATE	# WEEK	

NAME	🌿 DOSAGE	🕐 TIME
		: AM / PM
		: AM / PM
		: AM / PM
		: AM / PM
		: AM / PM
		: AM / PM
		: AM / PM
		: AM / PM
		: AM / PM
		: AM / PM
		: AM / PM
		: AM / PM
		: AM / PM
		: AM / PM
		: AM / PM

SIDE EFFECTS	📝 ADDITIONAL NOTES

PHYSICAL CONDITION		
SLEEP		WATER
ENERGY		ACTIVITY

📅 DATE		# WEEK

💊 NAME	🌱 DOSAGE	⏰ TIME
		: AM
		: AM
		: AM
		: AM
		: AM
		: AM
		: AM
		: AM
		: AM
		: AM
		: AM
		: AM
		: AM
		: AM
		: AM

🗣 SIDE EFFECTS	📝 ADDITIONAL NOTES
•	
•	
•	
•	
•	

PHYSICAL CONDITION

🌙 SLEEP		🥛 WATER	
⚡ ENERGY		🏃 ACTIVITY	

📅 DATE		#️⃣ WEEK

💊 NAME	🧪 DOSAGE	⏱️ TIME	
		:	AM / PM
		:	AM / PM
		:	AM / PM
		:	AM / PM
		:	AM / PM
		:	AM / PM
		:	AM / PM
		:	AM / PM
		:	AM / PM
		:	AM / PM
		:	AM / PM
		:	AM / PM
		:	AM / PM
		:	AM / PM
		:	AM / PM

🧠 SIDE EFFECTS

📝 ADDITIONAL NOTES

PHYSICAL CONDITION

🌙 SLEEP		🥛 WATER	
⚡ ENERGY		🏃 ACTIVITY	

📅 DATE		#️⃣ WEEK	

💊 NAME	🧪 DOSAGE	🕐 TIME	
		:	AM / P
		:	AM / P
		:	AM / P
		:	AM / P
		:	AM / P
		:	AM / P
		:	AM / P
		:	AM / P
		:	AM / P
		:	AM / P
		:	AM / P
		:	AM / P
		:	AM / P
		:	AM / P
		:	AM / P

🗣 SIDE EFFECTS	📝 ADDITIONAL NOTES
•	
•	
•	
•	
•	

PHYSICAL CONDITION	
🌙 SLEEP	💧 WATER
⚡ ENERGY	🏃 ACTIVITY

📆 DATE	# WEEK

💊 NAME	🧴 DOSAGE	⏰ TIME	
		:	AM / PM
		:	AM / PM
		:	AM / PM
		:	AM / PM
		:	AM / PM
		:	AM / PM
		:	AM / PM
		:	AM / PM
		:	AM / PM
		:	AM / PM
		:	AM / PM
		:	AM / PM
		:	AM / PM
		:	AM / PM

😷 SIDE EFFECTS	📝 ADDITIONAL NOTES

PHYSICAL CONDITION

🌙 SLEEP	▭▭▭▭▭	💧 WATER	▭▭▭▭▭
⚡ ENERGY	▭▭▭▭▭	🏃 ACTIVITY	▭▭▭▭▭

📅 DATE		#️⃣ WEEK

💊 NAME	🪴 DOSAGE	⏰ TIME
		: AM / P
		: AM / P
		: AM / P
		: AM / P
		: AM / P
		: AM / P
		: AM / P
		: AM / P
		: AM / P
		: AM / P
		: AM / P
		: AM / P
		: AM / P
		: AM / P
		: AM / P

🗣 SIDE EFFECTS	📝 ADDITIONAL NOTES
•	
•	
•	
•	
•	

PHYSICAL CONDITION

🌙 SLEEP	⬭⬭⬭⬭⬭	🥛 WATER	⬭⬭⬭⬭⬭
⚡ ENERGY	⬭⬭⬭⬭⬭	🏃 ACTIVITY	⬭⬭⬭⬭⬭

📅 DATE	# WEEK

💊 NAME	🌱 DOSAGE	⏱ TIME
		: AM / PM
		: AM / PM
		: AM / PM
		: AM / PM
		: AM / PM
		: AM / PM
		: AM / PM
		: AM / PM
		: AM / PM
		: AM / PM
		: AM / PM
		: AM / PM
		: AM / PM
		: AM / PM
		: AM / PM

🗣 SIDE EFFECTS	📝 ADDITIONAL NOTES

PHYSICAL CONDITION

🌙 SLEEP		🥛 WATER	
⚡ ENERGY		🏃 ACTIVITY	

📅 DATE		# WEEK

💊 NAME	🌱 DOSAGE	⏰ TIME
		: AM / P
		: AM / P
		: AM / P
		: AM / P
		: AM / P
		: AM / P
		: AM / P
		: AM / P
		: AM / P
		: AM / P
		: AM / P
		: AM / P
		: AM / P
		: AM / P
		: AM / P

🧠 SIDE EFFECTS	📝 ADDITIONAL NOTES
•	
•	
•	
•	
•	

PHYSICAL CONDITION	
🌙 SLEEP	🥤 WATER
⚡ ENERGY	🏃 ACTIVITY

DATE | **# WEEK**

NAME	DOSAGE	TIME
		: AM / PM
		: AM / PM
		: AM / PM
		: AM / PM
		: AM / PM
		: AM / PM
		: AM / PM
		: AM / PM
		: AM / PM
		: AM / PM
		: AM / PM
		: AM / PM
		: AM / PM
		: AM / PM
		: AM / PM

SIDE EFFECTS	ADDITIONAL NOTES

PHYSICAL CONDITION

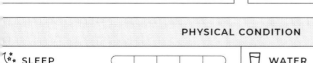

SLEEP | WATER

ENERGY | ACTIVITY

📅 DATE		#️⃣ WEEK	

💊 NAME	🌿 DOSAGE	⏰ TIME	
		:	AM / P
		:	AM / P
		:	AM / P
		:	AM / P
		:	AM / P
		:	AM / P
		:	AM / P
		:	AM / P
		:	AM / P
		:	AM / P
		:	AM / P
		:	AM / P
		:	AM / P
		:	AM / P
		:	AM / P

🧠 SIDE EFFECTS	📝 ADDITIONAL NOTES
•	
•	
•	
•	
•	

PHYSICAL CONDITION	
🌙 SLEEP	🥤 WATER
⚡ ENERGY	🏃 ACTIVITY

DATE	# WEEK

NAME	DOSAGE	TIME
		: AM / PM
		: AM / PM
		: AM / PM
		: AM / PM
		: AM / PM
		: AM / PM
		: AM / PM
		: AM / PM
		: AM / PM
		: AM / PM
		: AM / PM
		: AM / PM
		: AM / PM
		: AM / PM

SIDE EFFECTS	ADDITIONAL NOTES

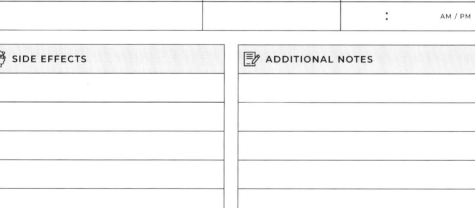

PHYSICAL CONDITION

SLEEP		WATER	
ENERGY		ACTIVITY	

📅 DATE		# WEEK

💊 NAME	🌱 DOSAGE	⏰ TIME
		: AM / P
		: AM / P
		: AM / P
		: AM / P
		: AM / P
		: AM / P
		: AM / P
		: AM / P
		: AM / P
		: AM / P
		: AM / P
		: AM / P
		: AM / P
		: AM / P
		: AM / P

🧠 SIDE EFFECTS	📝 ADDITIONAL NOTES
•	
•	
•	
•	
•	

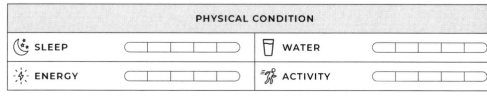

PHYSICAL CONDITION

🌙 SLEEP	⬜⬜⬜⬜⬜	🥛 WATER	⬜⬜⬜⬜⬜
⚡ ENERGY	⬜⬜⬜⬜⬜	🏃 ACTIVITY	⬜⬜⬜⬜⬜

📓 DATE		#️⃣ WEEK

💊 NAME	🌱 DOSAGE	⏰ TIME	
		:	AM / PM
		:	AM / PM
		:	AM / PM
		:	AM / PM
		:	AM / PM
		:	AM / PM
		:	AM / PM
		:	AM / PM
		:	AM / PM
		:	AM / PM
		:	AM / PM
		:	AM / PM
		:	AM / PM
		:	AM / PM

🗣 SIDE EFFECTS

📝 ADDITIONAL NOTES

PHYSICAL CONDITION

🌙 SLEEP		💧 WATER	
⚡ ENERGY		🏃 ACTIVITY	

📅 DATE		#️⃣ WEEK

💊 NAME	🪴 DOSAGE	💊 TIME	
		:	AM / P
		:	AM / P
		:	AM / P
		:	AM / P
		:	AM / P
		:	AM / P
		:	AM / P
		:	AM / P
		:	AM / P
		:	AM / P
		:	AM / P
		:	AM / P
		:	AM / P
		:	AM / P
		:	AM / P

🧠 SIDE EFFECTS

-
-
-
-
-

📝 ADDITIONAL NOTES

PHYSICAL CONDITION

🌙 SLEEP		💧 WATER	
⚡ ENERGY		🏃 ACTIVITY	

📋 DATE		# WEEK

🌱 NAME	💊 DOSAGE	🕐 TIME
		: AM / PM
		: AM / PM
		: AM / PM
		: AM / PM
		: AM / PM
		: AM / PM
		: AM / PM
		: AM / PM
		: AM / PM
		: AM / PM
		: AM / PM
		: AM / PM
		: AM / PM
		: AM / PM

🗣 SIDE EFFECTS	📝 ADDITIONAL NOTES

PHYSICAL CONDITION

🌙 SLEEP		🥛 WATER	
⚡ ENERGY		🏃 ACTIVITY	

📅 DATE		# WEEK	

💊 NAME	🌱 DOSAGE	⏰ TIME	
		:	AM / P
		:	AM / P
		:	AM / P
		:	AM / P
		:	AM / P
		:	AM / P
		:	AM / P
		:	AM / P
		:	AM / P
		:	AM / P
		:	AM / P
		:	AM / P
		:	AM / P
		:	AM / P
		:	AM / P

🗣 SIDE EFFECTS	📝 ADDITIONAL NOTES
•	
•	
•	
•	
•	

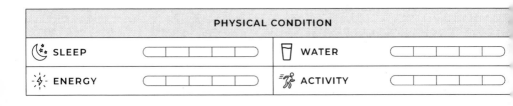

PHYSICAL CONDITION

🌙 SLEEP	▭▭▭▭▭	🥛 WATER	▭▭▭▭▭
⚡ ENERGY	▭▭▭▭▭	🏃 ACTIVITY	▭▭▭▭▭

DATE		# WEEK

NAME	DOSAGE	TIME	
		:	AM / PM
		:	AM / PM
		:	AM / PM
		:	AM / PM
		:	AM / PM
		:	AM / PM
		:	AM / PM
		:	AM / PM
		:	AM / PM
		:	AM / PM
		:	AM / PM
		:	AM / PM
		:	AM / PM
		:	AM / PM

SIDE EFFECTS	ADDITIONAL NOTES

PHYSICAL CONDITION

SLEEP		WATER	
ENERGY		ACTIVITY	

📅 DATE		# WEEK

💊 NAME	🌱 DOSAGE	🕐 TIME	
		:	AM / P
		:	AM / P
		:	AM / P
		:	AM / P
		:	AM / P
		:	AM / P
		:	AM / P
		:	AM / P
		:	AM / P
		:	AM / P
		:	AM / P
		:	AM / P
		:	AM / P
		:	AM / P
		:	AM / P

🧠 SIDE EFFECTS	📝 ADDITIONAL NOTES
•	
•	
•	
•	
•	

PHYSICAL CONDITION

🌙 SLEEP		💧 WATER	
⚡ ENERGY		🏃 ACTIVITY	

▤ DATE		# WEEK

◌ NAME	🌱 DOSAGE	🕐 TIME
		: AM / PM
		: AM / PM
		: AM / PM
		: AM / PM
		: AM / PM
		: AM / PM
		: AM / PM
		: AM / PM
		: AM / PM
		: AM / PM
		: AM / PM
		: AM / PM
		: AM / PM
		: AM / PM
		: AM / PM

😕 SIDE EFFECTS	📝 ADDITIONAL NOTES

PHYSICAL CONDITION	
🌙 SLEEP	🥛 WATER
⚡ ENERGY	🏃 ACTIVITY

📅 DATE		#️⃣ WEEK

💊 NAME	🌱 DOSAGE	⏰ TIME	
		:	AM / P
		:	AM / P
		:	AM / P
		:	AM / P
		:	AM / P
		:	AM / P
		:	AM / P
		:	AM / P
		:	AM / P
		:	AM / P
		:	AM / P
		:	AM / P
		:	AM / P
		:	AM / P
		:	AM / P

🧠 SIDE EFFECTS	📝 ADDITIONAL NOTES
•	
•	
•	
•	
•	

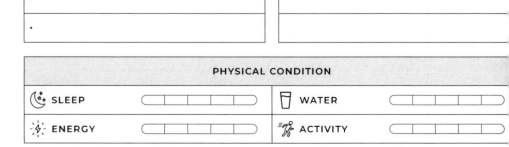

PHYSICAL CONDITION

🌙 SLEEP	🥛 WATER
⚡ ENERGY	🏃 ACTIVITY

▤ DATE	# WEEK

🧴 NAME	🧴 DOSAGE	💊 TIME	
		:	AM / PM
		:	AM / PM
		:	AM / PM
		:	AM / PM
		:	AM / PM
		:	AM / PM
		:	AM / PM
		:	AM / PM
		:	AM / PM
		:	AM / PM
		:	AM / PM
		:	AM / PM
		:	AM / PM
		:	AM / PM
		:	AM / PM

😣 SIDE EFFECTS	📝 ADDITIONAL NOTES

PHYSICAL CONDITION

🌙 SLEEP		🥛 WATER	
⚡ ENERGY		🏃 ACTIVITY	

📅 DATE		# WEEK

💊 NAME	🌱 DOSAGE	⏰ TIME
		: AM / P
		: AM / P
		: AM / P
		: AM / P
		: AM / P
		: AM / P
		: AM / P
		: AM / P
		: AM / P
		: AM / P
		: AM / P
		: AM / P
		: AM / P
		: AM / P
		: AM / P

🧠 SIDE EFFECTS

-
-
-
-
-

📝 ADDITIONAL NOTES

PHYSICAL CONDITION

🌙 SLEEP		💧 WATER	
⚡ ENERGY		🏃 ACTIVITY	

📅 DATE		#️⃣ WEEK

💊 NAME	🧪 DOSAGE	⏰ TIME
		: AM / PM
		: AM / PM
		: AM / PM
		: AM / PM
		: AM / PM
		: AM / PM
		: AM / PM
		: AM / PM
		: AM / PM
		: AM / PM
		: AM / PM
		: AM / PM
		: AM / PM
		: AM / PM

😣 SIDE EFFECTS	📝 ADDITIONAL NOTES

PHYSICAL CONDITION	
😴 SLEEP	💧 WATER
⚡ ENERGY	🏃 ACTIVITY

📅 DATE		# WEEK

💊 NAME	🌱 DOSAGE	⏰ TIME
		: AM / P
		: AM / P
		: AM / P
		: AM / P
		: AM / P
		: AM / P
		: AM / P
		: AM / P
		: AM / P
		: AM / P
		: AM / P
		: AM / P
		: AM / P
		: AM / P

🧠 SIDE EFFECTS	📝 ADDITIONAL NOTES
•	
•	
•	
•	
•	

PHYSICAL CONDITION

🌙 SLEEP		🥛 WATER	
⚡ ENERGY		🏃 ACTIVITY	

DATE	WEEK

NAME	DOSAGE	TIME
		: AM / PM
		: AM / PM
		: AM / PM
		: AM / PM
		: AM / PM
		: AM / PM
		: AM / PM
		: AM / PM
		: AM / PM
		: AM / PM
		: AM / PM
		: AM / PM
		: AM / PM
		: AM / PM
		: AM / PM

SIDE EFFECTS	ADDITIONAL NOTES

PHYSICAL CONDITION

SLEEP	WATER
ENERGY	ACTIVITY

📅 DATE		#️⃣ WEEK

💊 NAME	🌱 DOSAGE	⏰ TIME
		: AM / P
		: AM / P
		: AM / P
		: AM / P
		: AM / P
		: AM / P
		: AM / P
		: AM / P
		: AM / P
		: AM / P
		: AM / P
		: AM / P
		: AM / P
		: AM / P
		: AM / P

🧠 SIDE EFFECTS

-
-
-
-
-

📝 ADDITIONAL NOTES

PHYSICAL CONDITION

🌙 SLEEP		🥛 WATER	
⚡ ENERGY		🏃 ACTIVITY	

📅 DATE		# WEEK	

💊 NAME	🧪 DOSAGE	⏰ TIME	
		:	AM / PM
		:	AM / PM
		:	AM / PM
		:	AM / PM
		:	AM / PM
		:	AM / PM
		:	AM / PM
		:	AM / PM
		:	AM / PM
		:	AM / PM
		:	AM / PM
		:	AM / PM
		:	AM / PM
		:	AM / PM

🙂 SIDE EFFECTS	📝 ADDITIONAL NOTES

PHYSICAL CONDITION

🌙 SLEEP	⬜⬜⬜⬜⬜	💧 WATER	⬜⬜⬜⬜⬜
⚡ ENERGY	⬜⬜⬜⬜⬜	🏃 ACTIVITY	⬜⬜⬜⬜⬜

📅 DATE		#️⃣ WEEK

💊 NAME	💊 DOSAGE	⏰ TIME	
		:	AM / P
		:	AM / P
		:	AM / P
		:	AM / P
		:	AM / P
		:	AM / P
		:	AM / P
		:	AM / P
		:	AM / P
		:	AM / P
		:	AM / P
		:	AM / P
		:	AM / P
		:	AM / P
		:	AM / P

🧠 SIDE EFFECTS	📝 ADDITIONAL NOTES
.	
.	
.	
.	
.	

PHYSICAL CONDITION			
🌙 SLEEP		🥤 WATER	
⚡ ENERGY		🏃 ACTIVITY	

📅 DATE		#️⃣ WEEK	

🧫 NAME	🪴 DOSAGE	💊 TIME	
		:	AM / PM
		:	AM / PM
		:	AM / PM
		:	AM / PM
		:	AM / PM
		:	AM / PM
		:	AM / PM
		:	AM / PM
		:	AM / PM
		:	AM / PM
		:	AM / PM
		:	AM / PM
		:	AM / PM
		:	AM / PM
		:	AM / PM

🗣 SIDE EFFECTS	📝 ADDITIONAL NOTES

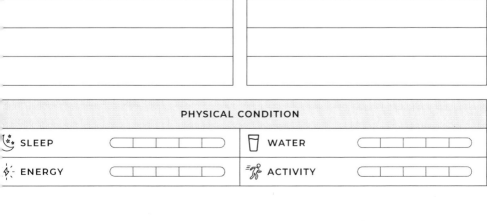

PHYSICAL CONDITION

✨ SLEEP		🥛 WATER	
⚡ ENERGY		🏃 ACTIVITY	

📅 DATE		#️⃣ WEEK

💊 NAME	🌱 DOSAGE	🕐 TIME
		: AM / P
		: AM / P
		: AM / P
		: AM / P
		: AM / P
		: AM / P
		: AM / P
		: AM / P
		: AM / P
		: AM / P
		: AM / P
		: AM / P
		: AM / P
		: AM / P
		: AM / P

🗣️ SIDE EFFECTS	📝 ADDITIONAL NOTES
•	
•	
•	
•	
•	

PHYSICAL CONDITION

🌙 SLEEP	☐☐☐☐☐	🥛 WATER	☐☐☐☐☐
⚡ ENERGY	☐☐☐☐☐	🏃 ACTIVITY	☐☐☐☐☐

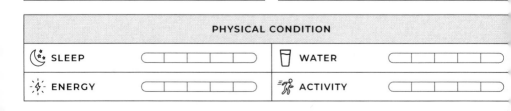

📅 DATE		# WEEK

💊 NAME	💊 DOSAGE	🕐 TIME
		: AM / PM
		: AM / PM
		: AM / PM
		: AM / PM
		: AM / PM
		: AM / PM
		: AM / PM
		: AM / PM
		: AM / PM
		: AM / PM
		: AM / PM
		: AM / PM
		: AM / PM
		: AM / PM
		: AM / PM

🗣 SIDE EFFECTS	📝 ADDITIONAL NOTES

PHYSICAL CONDITION

🌙 SLEEP	☐☐☐☐☐	🥛 WATER	☐☐☐☐☐
⚡ ENERGY	☐☐☐☐☐	🏃 ACTIVITY	☐☐☐☐☐

📅 DATE		#️⃣ WEEK

💊 NAME	💊 DOSAGE	🕐 TIME	
		:	AM / P
		:	AM / P
		:	AM / P
		:	AM / P
		:	AM / P
		:	AM / P
		:	AM / P
		:	AM / P
		:	AM / P
		:	AM / P
		:	AM / P
		:	AM / P
		:	AM / P
		:	AM / P
		:	AM / PM

🧠 SIDE EFFECTS	📝 ADDITIONAL NOTES
•	
•	
•	
•	
•	

PHYSICAL CONDITION			
🌙 SLEEP	▭▭▭▭▭	💧 WATER	▭▭▭▭▭
⚡ ENERGY	▭▭▭▭▭	🏃 ACTIVITY	▭▭▭▭▭

DATE		# WEEK	

👐 NAME	🌿 DOSAGE	🕐 TIME	
		:	AM / PM
		:	AM / PM
		:	AM / PM
		:	AM / PM
		:	AM / PM
		:	AM / PM
		:	AM / PM
		:	AM / PM
		:	AM / PM
		:	AM / PM
		:	AM / PM
		:	AM / PM
		:	AM / PM
		:	AM / PM

😣 SIDE EFFECTS	📝 ADDITIONAL NOTES

PHYSICAL CONDITION

🌙 SLEEP		🥛 WATER	
⚡ ENERGY		🏃 ACTIVITY	

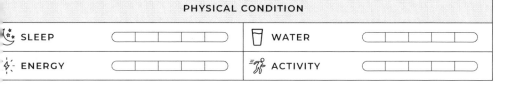

📅 DATE		# WEEK	

💊 NAME	🌿 DOSAGE	🕐 TIME	
		:	AM / P
		:	AM / P
		:	AM / P
		:	AM / P
		:	AM / P
		:	AM / P
		:	AM / P
		:	AM / P
		:	AM / P
		:	AM / P
		:	AM / P
		:	AM / P
		:	AM / P
		:	AM / P
		:	AM / P

🧠 SIDE EFFECTS	📝 ADDITIONAL NOTES
•	
•	
•	
•	
•	

PHYSICAL CONDITION

🌙 SLEEP	⬜⬜⬜⬜⬜	🥛 WATER	⬜⬜⬜⬜⬜
⚡ ENERGY	⬜⬜⬜⬜⬜	🏃 ACTIVITY	⬜⬜⬜⬜⬜

DATE	# WEEK

🧬 NAME	🌱 DOSAGE	🕐 TIME
		: AM / PM
		: AM / PM
		: AM / PM
		: AM / PM
		: AM / PM
		: AM / PM
		: AM / PM
		: AM / PM
		: AM / PM
		: AM / PM
		: AM / PM
		: AM / PM
		: AM / PM
		: AM / PM
		: AM / PM

😖 SIDE EFFECTS	📝 ADDITIONAL NOTES

PHYSICAL CONDITION

🌙 SLEEP	▭▭▭▭▭	🥛 WATER	▭▭▭▭▭
⚡ ENERGY	▭▭▭▭▭	🏃 ACTIVITY	▭▭▭▭▭

📅 DATE		# WEEK

💊 NAME	💊 DOSAGE	⏰ TIME
		: AM / P
		: AM / P
		: AM / P
		: AM / P
		: AM / P
		: AM / P
		: AM / P
		: AM / P
		: AM / P
		: AM / P
		: AM / P
		: AM / P
		: AM / P
		: AM / P
		: AM / P

🧠 SIDE EFFECTS	📝 ADDITIONAL NOTES
•	
•	
•	
•	
•	

PHYSICAL CONDITION

🌙 SLEEP	☐☐☐☐☐	🥛 WATER	☐☐☐☐☐
⚡ ENERGY	☐☐☐☐☐	🏃 ACTIVITY	☐☐☐☐☐

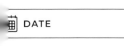 **DATE** | **WEEK**

🧪 NAME	🪴 DOSAGE	⏰ TIME
		: AM / PM
		: AM / PM
		: AM / PM
		: AM / PM
		: AM / PM
		: AM / PM
		: AM / PM
		: AM / PM
		: AM / PM
		: AM / PM
		: AM / PM
		: AM / PM
		: AM / PM
		: AM / PM
		: AM / PM

🧠 SIDE EFFECTS	📝 ADDITIONAL NOTES

PHYSICAL CONDITION

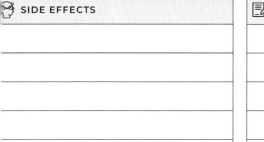

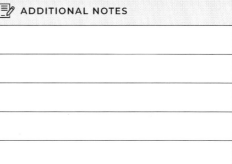

🌙 SLEEP   ☐☐☐☐☐   🥤 WATER   ☐☐☐☐☐

⚡ ENERGY   ☐☐☐☐☐   🏃 ACTIVITY   ☐☐☐☐☐

📅 DATE		#️⃣ WEEK

💊 NAME	🌱 DOSAGE	🕐 TIME
		: AM / P
		: AM / P
		: AM / P
		: AM / P
		: AM / P
		: AM / P
		: AM / P
		: AM / P
		: AM / P
		: AM / P
		: AM / P
		: AM / P
		: AM / P
		: AM / P
		: AM / P

🧠 SIDE EFFECTS	📝 ADDITIONAL NOTES
•	
•	
•	
•	
•	

PHYSICAL CONDITION	
🌙 SLEEP	🥛 WATER
⚡ ENERGY	🏃 ACTIVITY

📓 DATE	# WEEK

💊 NAME	💊 DOSAGE	🕐 TIME
		: AM / PM
		: AM / PM
		: AM / PM
		: AM / PM
		: AM / PM
		: AM / PM
		: AM / PM
		: AM / PM
		: AM / PM
		: AM / PM
		: AM / PM
		: AM / PM
		: AM / PM
		: AM / PM
		: AM / PM

🧠 SIDE EFFECTS	📝 ADDITIONAL NOTES

PHYSICAL CONDITION

🌙 SLEEP	🔲🔲🔲🔲	🥛 WATER	🔲🔲🔲🔲
⚡ ENERGY	🔲🔲🔲🔲	🏃 ACTIVITY	🔲🔲🔲🔲

📅 DATE		#️⃣ WEEK	

💊 NAME	🌱 DOSAGE	🕐 TIME	
		:	AM / P
		:	AM / P
		:	AM / P
		:	AM / P
		:	AM / P
		:	AM / P
		:	AM / P
		:	AM / P
		:	AM / P
		:	AM / P
		:	AM / P
		:	AM / P
		:	AM / P
		:	AM / P

🧠 SIDE EFFECTS	📝 ADDITIONAL NOTES
•	
•	
•	
•	
•	

PHYSICAL CONDITION

🌙 SLEEP		🥛 WATER	
⚡ ENERGY		🏃 ACTIVITY	

📓 DATE		#⃞ WEEK	

💊 NAME	🪴 DOSAGE	🕐 TIME	
		:	AM / PM
		:	AM / PM
		:	AM / PM
		:	AM / PM
		:	AM / PM
		:	AM / PM
		:	AM / PM
		:	AM / PM
		:	AM / PM
		:	AM / PM
		:	AM / PM
		:	AM / PM
		:	AM / PM
		:	AM / PM

😁 SIDE EFFECTS	📝 ADDITIONAL NOTES

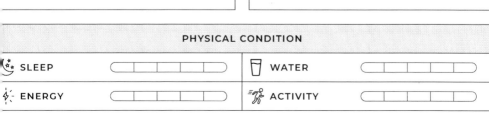

PHYSICAL CONDITION

🌙 SLEEP	▭▭▭▭▭	🥛 WATER	▭▭▭▭▭
⚡ ENERGY	▭▭▭▭▭	🏃 ACTIVITY	▭▭▭▭▭

📅 DATE	#️⃣ WEEK

💊 NAME	💊 DOSAGE	⏰ TIME
		: AM / P
		: AM / P
		: AM / P
		: AM / P
		: AM / P
		: AM / P
		: AM / P
		: AM / P
		: AM / P
		: AM / P
		: AM / P
		: AM / P
		: AM / P
		: AM / P

🗣 SIDE EFFECTS	📝 ADDITIONAL NOTES
•	
•	
•	
•	
•	

PHYSICAL CONDITION

🌙 SLEEP		🥛 WATER	
⚡ ENERGY		🏃 ACTIVITY	

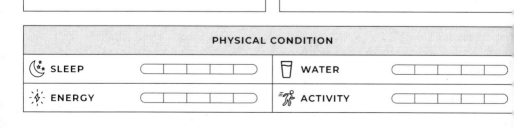

📓 DATE		#️⃣ WEEK

💊 NAME	🧪 DOSAGE	🕐 TIME
		: AM / PM
		: AM / PM
		: AM / PM
		: AM / PM
		: AM / PM
		: AM / PM
		: AM / PM
		: AM / PM
		: AM / PM
		: AM / PM
		: AM / PM
		: AM / PM
		: AM / PM
		: AM / PM
		: AM / PM

🧠 SIDE EFFECTS

📝 ADDITIONAL NOTES

PHYSICAL CONDITION

🌙 SLEEP   ⬚⬚⬚⬚⬚   💧 WATER   ⬚⬚⬚⬚⬚

⚡ ENERGY   ⬚⬚⬚⬚⬚   🏃 ACTIVITY   ⬚⬚⬚⬚⬚

📅 DATE		#️⃣ WEEK

💊 NAME	🌱 DOSAGE	💊 TIME
		: AM / P
		: AM / P
		: AM / P
		: AM / P
		: AM / P
		: AM / P
		: AM / P
		: AM / P
		: AM / P
		: AM / P
		: AM / P
		: AM / P
		: AM / P
		: AM / P
		: AM / P

🧠 SIDE EFFECTS	📝 ADDITIONAL NOTES
•	
•	
•	
•	
•	

PHYSICAL CONDITION	
🌙 SLEEP	🥛 WATER
⚡ ENERGY	🏃 ACTIVITY

📓 DATE		#️⃣ WEEK

🧪 NAME	💊 DOSAGE	⏰ TIME
		: AM / PM
		: AM / PM
		: AM / PM
		: AM / PM
		: AM / PM
		: AM / PM
		: AM / PM
		: AM / PM
		: AM / PM
		: AM / PM
		: AM / PM
		: AM / PM
		: AM / PM
		: AM / PM

😕 SIDE EFFECTS	📝 ADDITIONAL NOTES

PHYSICAL CONDITION

🌙 SLEEP		🥛 WATER	
⚡ ENERGY		🏃 ACTIVITY	

📅 DATE		#️⃣ WEEK

💊 NAME	🌱 DOSAGE	🕐 TIME
		: AM / P
		: AM / P
		: AM / P
		: AM / P
		: AM / P
		: AM / P
		: AM / P
		: AM / P
		: AM / P
		: AM / P
		: AM / P
		: AM / P
		: AM / P
		: AM / P
		: AM / P

🧠 SIDE EFFECTS	📝 ADDITIONAL NOTES
•	
•	
•	
•	
•	

PHYSICAL CONDITION

🌙 SLEEP	⬜⬜⬜⬜⬜	🥤 WATER	⬜⬜⬜⬜⬜
⚡ ENERGY	⬜⬜⬜⬜⬜	🏃 ACTIVITY	⬜⬜⬜⬜⬜

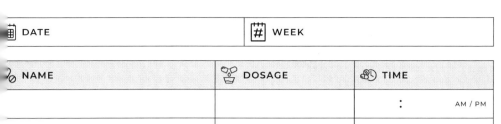

DATE	# WEEK

🖊 NAME	💊 DOSAGE	⏰ TIME	
		:	AM / PM
		:	AM / PM
		:	AM / PM
		:	AM / PM
		:	AM / PM
		:	AM / PM
		:	AM / PM
		:	AM / PM
		:	AM / PM
		:	AM / PM
		:	AM / PM
		:	AM / PM
		:	AM / PM
		:	AM / PM

🧠 SIDE EFFECTS	📝 ADDITIONAL NOTES

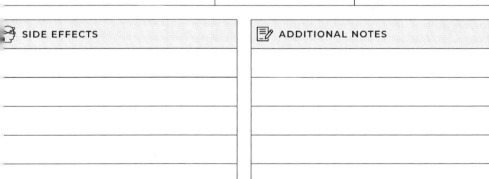

PHYSICAL CONDITION

🌙 SLEEP		🥛 WATER	
⚡ ENERGY		🏃 ACTIVITY	

📅 DATE		# WEEK

💊 NAME	💊 DOSAGE	🕐 TIME
		: AM / P
		: AM / P
		: AM / P
		: AM / P
		: AM / P
		: AM / P
		: AM / P
		: AM / P
		: AM / P
		: AM / P
		: AM / P
		: AM / P
		: AM / P
		: AM / P
		: AM / PM

🗣 SIDE EFFECTS	📝 ADDITIONAL NOTES
•	
•	
•	
•	
•	

PHYSICAL CONDITION

🌙 SLEEP	▭▭▭▭▭	🥛 WATER	▭▭▭▭▭
⚡ ENERGY	▭▭▭▭▭	🏃 ACTIVITY	▭▭▭▭▭

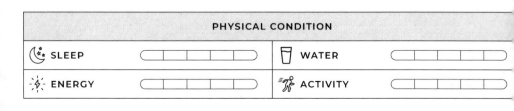

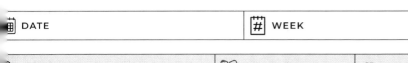

📅 DATE		# WEEK

💊 NAME	💊 DOSAGE	🕐 TIME
		: AM / PM
		: AM / PM
		: AM / PM
		: AM / PM
		: AM / PM
		: AM / PM
		: AM / PM
		: AM / PM
		: AM / PM
		: AM / PM
		: AM / PM
		: AM / PM
		: AM / PM
		: AM / PM
		: AM / PM

🧠 SIDE EFFECTS	📝 ADDITIONAL NOTES

PHYSICAL CONDITION

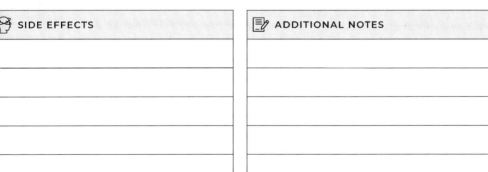

🌙 SLEEP		🥤 WATER	
⚡ ENERGY		🏃 ACTIVITY	

🗓 DATE		# WEEK	

💊 NAME	🌱 DOSAGE	🕐 TIME	
		:	AM / P
		:	AM / P
		:	AM / P
		:	AM / P
		:	AM / P
		:	AM / P
		:	AM / P
		:	AM / P
		:	AM / P
		:	AM / P
		:	AM / P
		:	AM / P
		:	AM / P
		:	AM / P

🧠 SIDE EFFECTS	📝 ADDITIONAL NOTES
•	
•	
•	
•	
•	

PHYSICAL CONDITION	
🌙 SLEEP	🥤 WATER
⚡ ENERGY	🏃 ACTIVITY

DATE	**#** WEEK

🌱 NAME	🌱 DOSAGE	🕐 TIME
		: AM / PM
		: AM / PM
		: AM / PM
		: AM / PM
		: AM / PM
		: AM / PM
		: AM / PM
		: AM / PM
		: AM / PM
		: AM / PM
		: AM / PM
		: AM / PM
		: AM / PM
		: AM / PM
		: AM / PM

🙂 SIDE EFFECTS	📝 ADDITIONAL NOTES

PHYSICAL CONDITION

🌙 SLEEP		🥛 WATER	
⚡ ENERGY		🏃 ACTIVITY	

📅 DATE		#️⃣ WEEK

💊 NAME	🪴 DOSAGE	💊 TIME
		: AM / P
		: AM / P
		: AM / P
		: AM / P
		: AM / P
		: AM / P
		: AM / P
		: AM / P
		: AM / P
		: AM / P
		: AM / P
		: AM / P
		: AM / P
		: AM / P
		: AM / P

🧠 SIDE EFFECTS	📝 ADDITIONAL NOTES
•	
•	
•	
•	
•	

PHYSICAL CONDITION

🌙 SLEEP	▭▭▭▭▭	🥛 WATER	▭▭▭▭▭
⚡ ENERGY	▭▭▭▭▭	🏃 ACTIVITY	▭▭▭▭▭

Made in United States
Troutdale, OR
12/23/2024

27203922R00058